BEI GRIN MACHT SICH IHR WISSEN BEZAHLT

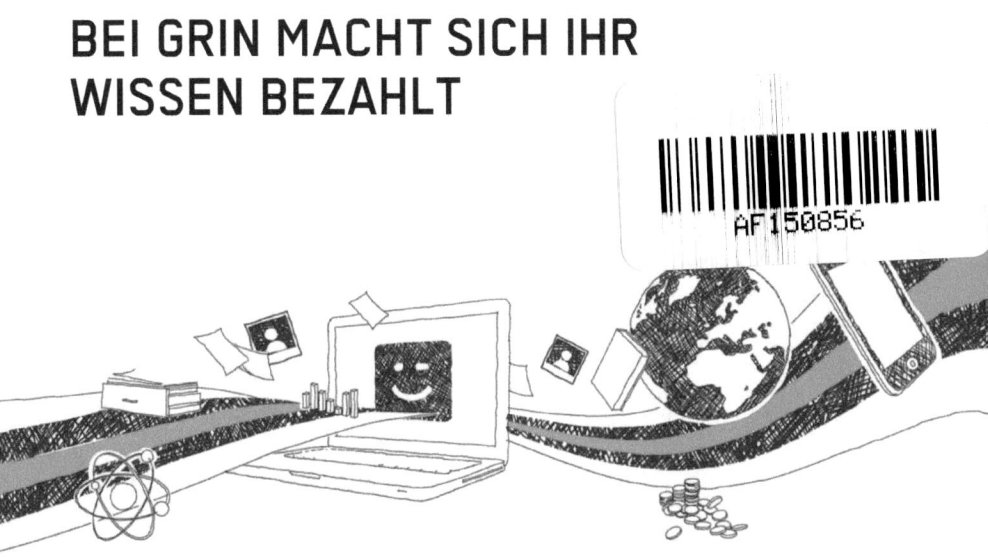

- Wir veröffentlichen Ihre Hausarbeit,
  Bachelor- und Masterarbeit

- Ihr eigenes eBook und Buch -
  weltweit in allen wichtigen Shops

- Verdienen Sie an jedem Verkauf

Jetzt bei www.GRIN.com hochladen und kostenlos publizieren

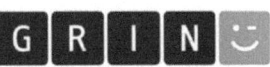

Bibliografische Information der Deutschen Nationalbibliothek:

Die Deutsche Bibliothek verzeichnet diese Publikation in der Deutschen National-
bibliografie; detaillierte bibliografische Daten sind im Internet über http://dnb.d-
nb.de/ abrufbar.

Impressum:

Copyright © 2017 GRIN Verlag, Open Publishing GmbH
Druck und Bindung: Books on Demand GmbH, Norderstedt Germany
ISBN: 9783668540248

Dieses Buch bei GRIN:

http://www.grin.com/de/e-book/376100/maintenance-of-facilities-a-study-of-the-
sanitation-facilities-in-public

Sally Koech

Maintenance of Facilities. A Study of the Sanitation Facilities in Public Primary School in Kericho Municipality

GRIN Verlag

GRIN - Your knowledge has value

Der GRIN Verlag publiziert seit 1998 wissenschaftliche Arbeiten von Studenten, Hochschullehrern und anderen Akademikern als eBook und gedrucktes Buch. Die Verlagswebsite www.grin.com ist die ideale Plattform zur Veröffentlichung von Hausarbeiten, Abschlussarbeiten, wissenschaftlichen Aufsätzen, Dissertationen und Fachbüchern.

Besuchen Sie uns im Internet:

http://www.grin.com/

http://www.facebook.com/grincom

http://www.twitter.com/grin_com

AN ASSESSMENT OF THE MAINTENANCE OF SANITATION FACILITIES IN KERICHO MUNICIPALITY, KERICHO COUNTY

Sally Cherono Koech, Department of Education Administration, University of Kabianga

ABSTRACT

Sanitation is a basic human right as ratified by most countries of the world in convection to the rights of a child (CRC) which states that children have a right to a safe environment that enhance learning, health and development of good citizens. The purpose of the study therefore was to assess the state of hygiene and maintenance of sanitation facilities and to determine if there were any differences in sanitation facilities per gender in public primary schools in Kericho Municipality. Survey research design was used to assess sanitation facilities in public primary schools. The target population comprised of all standard seven pupils in seventeen (17) public primary schools in Kericho Municipality. A stratified random sampling technique was applied to obtain a sample of 292 standard seven pupils from 5 public primary schools. The sample comprised of 147 boys and 145 girls. Data was collected using questionnaire and observation checklists. The questionnaire was used to collect data from pupils while observation schedules were used by the researcher to collect data from the schools. Data was analysed using frequencies, percentages, means and pie charts. The study concluded that the standard of maintenance of the sanitary facilities was below standard. Most facilities were in need of repair. The study recommended that the Ministry of Education should ensure that sanitation facilities meet National Standards and that these facilities are maintained in a regular manner. It is hoped that the study will lead to the improvement of sanitation facilities in public primary schools. The findings of this research will also assist the schools under study in planning, organizing and managing school sanitation facilities.

Keywords: *Maintenance, sanitation facilities*

Introduction

The health, academic performance and retention rates of school going children is adversely affected by availability accessibility and quality of stimuli facilitation. Studies indicate that 400 million children have diminished learning abilities due to intestinal worm infestation (Hall et al, 2008). On the other hand, according to international research centre on water and sanitation (IRC, 2005) 75 percent of adolescent girls drop out of school due to lack of adequate private sanitation facilities in school. The school environment represents an important setting because many children's social habits and behaviors are learned at school (United Nations (UN) (2011). However, availability of sanitation facilities is a fundamental and indisputable component of the teaching and learning process. In which the learner would exploit and maximize potential for learning. Since inadequate sanitation facilities make it difficult for pupils to concentrate, and for teachers to teach efficiently, which has been caused by failure to comply with the health and safety standards guidelines Health related problems are also reported due to poor school sanitation facilities such as diarrhea, worm infestation; typhoid which leads to student discomfort and psychological stress.

Health is compromised in a dirty and worn out sanitation facility, unventilated toilets, and broken doors, where pupils may be prone to disease such as cholera and diarrhea. The hygienic management of human excretes refuse and waste water, the control of disease vectors and provision of washing facilities for personal and domestic hygiene is essential so as to avoid water borne diseases as cholera and typhoid (UNICEF 2010).

The quality of the school shapes the attitude of teachers and learners whereby their attitude affects the learning behavior and performance. Blumende (2001) adds that decline in quality of education cannot be ignored by anyone as education is an instrument to societal transformation and development. It's through good interpersonal relationships in schools that good teaching and learning processes be achieved so that orphans, those with disabilities and those with special needs are catered for.

Statement of the Problem

With the introduction of Free Primary Education by the Kenyan Government in 2003, many challenges have been experienced such as; over stretched learning facilities, overcrowding in schools, high costs of equipment for the special needs leading to internal inefficiency making the school sanitation facilities strained UNICEF (2004). Although policy intervention vary depending on the setting, countries have been facing challenges in scaling up worldwide policies and sustaining policy intervention with limited budgets (Oseji and Okolo, 2011; WHO, 2011). A look at the government policies and publication does not indicate budgetary allocations made to maintain infrastructure provision or maintenance. The safety standards manual (2009) replaced the Ministry of Education circular (2001) that previously defined health and safety standards in educational institutions. This study therefore systematically assessed the sanitation facilities in public primary schools in Kericho Municipality. This study may therefore lead to the improvement of sanitation facilities. It may also form a base on which, other scholars can develop their studies. The findings of this research may also assist the schools under study in planning, organizing and managing school sanitation facilities. It may further help the schools to bench mark current policies and practices against current legislative requirements and best practices. It may help schools to meet legal obligation under sanitation facilities at work (Act, 2005). International guidelines on sanitation facilities government policies, National Health Policy MOPH / IMSE, 2009.

LITERATURE REVIEW

School WASH interventions are to improve overall sanitation, hygiene and daily water intake in both educational and non-educational environments. Many children in both developing and developed nations spend time absent from schools due to diseases contracted within the school environment United Nations UN, (2011). In which Minds 2006 concurs that in 2002, a national survey of urban schools teachers, 26% of Chicago teachers and more than 30 % of Washington DC teachers, reported health related problems due to poor school sanitation facility. However this study will look into hygiene and maintenance of sanitation in public primary schools in Kenya.

The international bodies as UNICEF, WHO among others have been active in spear heading, WASH campaigns across the world especially developing countries like Asia and Africa. Studies indicate that 272 million schools days are lost by children due to diarrhea annually (Hutton et al, 2004). This has great impact on academic performance. The availability of water and sanitation facilities in schools have reduce diarrhea and hygiene related diseases amongst school going children (Curtis et al; 2003; Pruss et al, 2008)

Studies from the developing world indicate that 100% of annual soil transmitted worm infestation cases are attributed by inadequate sanitation and hygiene (Hall et al, 2008). This is has shown to be a cause of death for 1.8 people annually (WHO, 2010) whom most of them are from developing countries. The school environment is an important sector to explore due to the social and health influences schools have on children. In addition, the school environment is important for interventions aimed at mitigating infectious diseases spread because children may be introduced to more and more strains of pathogens in the school, due to the fact that more children are present in contact with and using the facilities. This exposure makes the school environment efficacious for performing. Greene et al, (2012) these then affects the pupils' participation leading to psychological instability which this study will explore.

Rukunga and Mutethia (2006), opines that school hygiene and sanitation education are areas of concern in as far as promotion of hygiene and sanitation act are concerned. This is because it would lead to pupil absenteeism from school due to common preventable diseases such as diarrhea. Sanitation facilities are therefore fundamental for promoting hygiene and proper behavior which would enhance good participation on state of sanitation facilities.

The aim of Universal Primary Education (U.P.E) is to ensure that all Kenyan children eligible for primary school have opportunity to enroll and remain in school to learn and acquire quality basic education and skills. The Kenyan government introduced F.P.E in 2003 which increased enrollment of children from 5.9 million in 2002 to 7.2 million in formal schools alone (Sessional paper No 1 of 2005). This has equally led to strained physical infrastructure.

The Kenyan government finance instructional materials but has left the task of building and maintaining to the parents who seem reluctant to pay thus leading to strained sanitation facilities in place. As such, overcrowded sanitation facilities lead to less interaction and poor participation. However, F.P.E has exacerbated these conditions. It is for this reason that inadequate sanitation further leads to stress, absenteeism and low self-esteem (WHO, 2010).

The magnitude of challenge has been underscored by WHO which ascribes that 80% of all sickness and diseases is due to lack of drinking water and sanitation leading to diarrhea, cholera, malaria among others.

In Senegal pupils avoid school toilet use as they associate it with immorality and dangers such as presence of snakes, filth concentration, rapes and drug exchange. This shows the extent to which fear and psychological discomfort pupils have towards the state of sanitation facilities which this study will look into.

Equally in Africa there was a case in Lesotho where pupils were assaulted and bullied each other Brener, Lowry & Barrios, (2005). Further, many reasons to complain of low performance was noted such as poor hygiene practices among school children lack of safe drinking water, and absenteeism being high. Pupils would go back to their homes to drink water and use toilets and not return; as such there were high dropout rates. There is a positive correlation between education quality of life, good health and economic activity. Studies indicates that 50 % of child mortality in Uganda is due to poor hygiene and sanitation children being susceptible UNICEF / SIDA, (2002). Schools like the rest of Uganda's infrastructure suffered a great deal of devastation during the 1970 and 1980 wars and political Upheaval .

However water and sanitation is below desired standards, only 29% of schools in the country have access to water and sanitary facilities. Where the MOEST (2003), rates Kenya in dangerous category where over 90% of primary schools in rural Kenya lack safe water and even the water needed for hand washing. Lack of separate toilets for maturing girls leads to frustration and ridicule by others thus imparting negatively on their perception of sanitation facilities. Sometime this leads to children having negative imagination on the toilets as they are filthy, congested, full of excrete and they are few. Such sanitation facilities lead to high incidence of diseases such as; worm infestation, typhoid or diarrhea. Indeed the environment of a child influences learning. WSP (2007) sanitation facilities have been cited as a factor that can push children particularly out of school, Water aid (2009). This claim has been supported by water and sanitation practitioners and organization. Lilonde, (2004) has written that poor sanitation limits attendance school dropouts and low literacy rates.

Hand washing with soap effectively reduces exposure to diarrhea-causing pathogens. Interventions to improve hygiene and sanitation conditions in schools within low-income countries have gained increased attention; however, their impact on schoolchildren's exposure to fecal pathogens has not been established (Greene, et al, 2012). This greatly affects on performance and retention of pupils.

A Study carried out in rural western Kenya showed that when children are actively engaged in WASH they lead to community adoption of good hygiene behaviors, leading to improved individual and community health (Gisore, 2013). This study assessed the hygiene and maintenance practices towards sanitation in public primary schools in Kericho Municipality.

RESARCH METHODOLOGY

The Research Design

A survey research was used in this study. This design was used to determine reasons or causes for the current status of the phenomenon under study. As a result of the cause-and-effect relationships, this research design does not permit manipulation of the variables (Patton, 2002). The design was adopted in this study because the cause, i.e. the independent variables was studied after they have exerted the effect on the dependent variable.

The study was conducted in Kericho County which is located south west of the Kenyan Rift Valley region. It lies between 35^0 -40^0 and latitude of 023^0 South East between the Equator. Kericho County has a population of 758,339 according to 2009 census. The county comprises of six sub counties or constituencies namely: Kipkelion East and West, Ainamoi, Belgut, Sigowet, Soin and Buret. Most of the activities in Kericho are agricultural as it has adequate rainfall.It is one of the leading country's tea exporters with high concentration of tea factories. It has a number of multinational tea companies among others. Ainamoi constituency has seven educational administrative zones namely; Municipality, Soin, Soliat, Ainamoi, Kapsaos and Koitaburot. The primary enrolment is 163,133. Teacher –pupil ration is 1: 33 public primary schools.

Kericho Municipality where the study was based is a cosmopolitan town and has realized a great influx of learners because it is a business centre which has several business people who have come to settle there. As such, there are a high number of learners in the schools leading to strained sanitation facilities. There are also many people who have come to settle in Kericho because of their interest in employment in the tea industry. The choice of Kericho municipality is because of the high population of pupils it holds. Since there is minimal research that has been done in this county, it is therefore believed that the findings of this study will be of use to Educational Planners.

Target Population

The target population for this study was standard seven pupils in seventeen (17) public primary schools in Kericho Municipality. Public primary schools were chosen because they are the ones who implement the ministry's policy and are funded by the government. They also have a large enrollment. Class seven pupils were preferred not only because of their long stay but because they were also able to understand the items in questions easily and respond to them. Class eight pupils were left out because they were preparing for KCPE examination.

Sample Size and Sampling Procedures

A sample is a set of respondents (people) selected from a larger population for the purpose of a convenience sampling. First, simple random sampling was used to select five (5) schools from the target population of seventeen (17) schools. Thereafter stratified random sampling technique was used to select a sample of 292 respondents comprising of 147 boys and 145 girls. Sample size determination is shown in Table 3.1;

Table 3.1

Sample size per school and category

School	Boys Total	Boys Sample	Girls Total	Girls Sample	Total Respondents	%
1. Highlands primary school	160	48	180	54	102	30%
2. St. Patricks primary school	90	27	96	28	55	30%
3. Chepkolon primary school	40	12	42	13	25	30%
4. Kimugu primary school	160	48	120	36	84	30%
5. Chelimo primary school	40	12	45	14	26	30%
Total	**565**	**147**	**532**	**145**	**292**	**30%**

Source: District Education Office, Kericho, 2016.

Data Collection Instruments

The researcher used questionnaires and observation checklists as the tools and instruments of data collection. The format for both questionnaire and observation checklist was developed using the Health Safety Manual Standards for schools in Kenya, MOE (2009) as a guiding document.

Data Collection Procedures

A letter of introduction from University of Kabianga was used to get a permit from NACOSTI. The researcher made a visit to the Sub County Director of Education to brief the officer about the research and to obtain a permission to undertake the study in the sub county. The researcher proceeded to each school in the sample to meet the head teacher and to explain the purpose of the research. The researcher administered the questionnaire to the pupils with the aid of their class teacher. The researcher utilized the observation checklist to record the adequacy of sanitation facilities, hygiene and maintenance of sanitation facilities as in appendix v.

Data Analysis and Presentations

Each data piece was inspected to determine its usefulness. Incomplete data pieces were discarded. Data cleaning was done prior to analysis. The researcher proceeded to summarize the data by objective. Data for objectives (i) to (iv) were analysed by use of frequencies, percentages and means. The results of the analysis were presented by use of tables, pie charts and figures. The findings of data analysis are discussed in chapter four.

Ethical Considerations

Ethical issues were considered such as, objectivity versus subjectivity was considered. So that his/her own biases and opinions do not get in the research. Moreover, the researcher kept the findings of this study confidential. The researcher sought permission from the primary schools indicated for the purpose of data collection. The researcher promised not reveal the collected data to any unauthorized persons. For purpose of privacy, their consent was sought if the information needed to be revealed and for confidentiality purposes. Moreover, the respondents were not revealed in any way so as to guard their privacy and enable them give information without fear. The researcher on the other hand, accepts any errors due to common errors or omission while compiling the report of this study.

RESULTS

Table 1: State of toilets as rated by boys and girls

	Boys		Girls	
	Frequency	**Percentage**	**Frequency**	**Percentage**
Poor	167	73.2	147	64.5
Fair	51	22.4	63	27.6
Good	10	4.4	18	7.9
Total	**228**	**100**	**228**	**100**

Source: Survey Data

Table 4.6 shows that majority of the boys' toilets 167 (73.2%) were in poor state compared to girls which 147 (64.5%). The finding is in line with the report of Kimani (2015) on state of latrines in Nakuru, which reported that many of the schools depicted a sorry state of the toilets, with many on the verge of collapsing while in some cases there were no toilets at all forcing children to use the bushes.

The findings also agree with the researcher's observation which noted that the state of the toilets were almost full in some cases, boys used behind the toilet instead of inside because of the poor state of the toilets. They were very dirty in some cases with feces scattered while in some there were no doors.

The boys were asked to rate the state of their urinals. The results of data analysis are indicated in Figure 4.3:

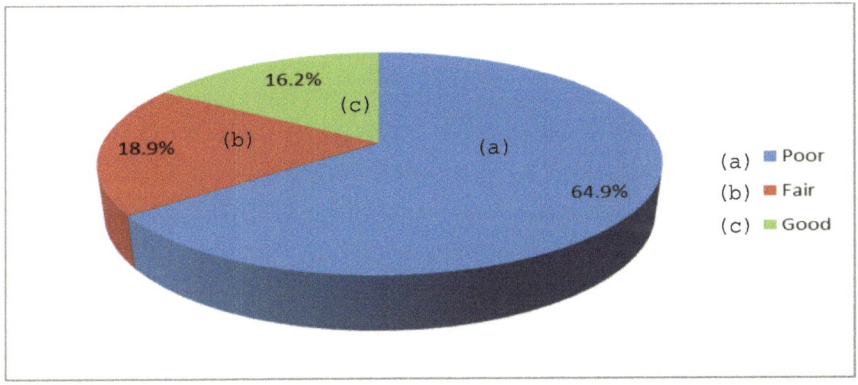

11

Figure 1: State of urinals as rated by boys and girls

Figure 1 reveals that majority of boys 64.9% rated the state of their urinals as poor. This is in line with the findings of Kwakye (2013) who established that majority of the schools studied had urinal and toilet but not enough to meet up the number of pupils found in the school and 23.5% had the facilities but were in a deplorable state.

The findings also agree with the researcher's observation which revealed that the urinals were in very poor state.

The girls were asked to rate the status of bathroom and the results are displayed in Figure 4.4.

Figure 2: State of bathrooms as rated by girls

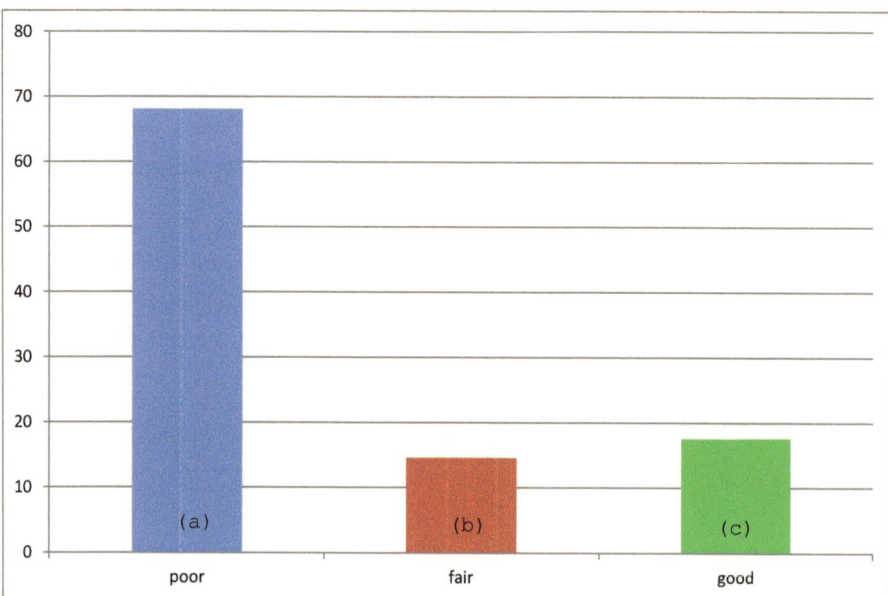

Figure 2. shows that the majority of the girls 155 (68%) rated the state of their bathrooms as poor. The findings revealed that bathrooms were unavailable in most of the schools studied which may contribute to absenteeism among the adolescent girls. According to WATER AID (2013), adolescent girls require access to menstrual hygiene management facilities in school. Girls often have to stay at home if they are unable to manage menstruation safely or with dignity. As a result, their academic performance is affected and many girls drop out of school permanently.

Table 2: State of hand washing points as rated respondents

	Frequency	Percentage
Poor	155	68
Fair	34	14.9
Good	39	17.1
Total	**228**	**100**

Source: Researcher 2016

Table 2 reveals that the majority 68% of the girls rated handwashing points as poor. According to Mbula (2013), schools, particularly those in rural areas often have inadequate water, toilets, hand washing with soap and hand washing facilities making it difficult for some students to practice proper hygiene. Boys and girls are likely to be affected in different ways by this inadequacy and this may contribute to unequal learning opportunities.

The observations made revealed the handwashing points were very muddy with long queues because the points were very few in majority of the schools.

The respondents were asked to rate the state of drinking points in their schools. The results are displayed in Table 3.

Table 3: State of drinking points as rated by respondents

	Frequency	Percentage
Poor	136	59.6
Fair	92	40.4
Total	**228**	**100**

Source: Researcher 2016

Table 3 shows that the majority 136 (59.6%) of the respondents rated the status of drinking points as poor. The findings concur with the findings of Barasa *et.al* which established that drinking water containers in majority of schools in Kakamega did not have a functioning taps while according to the National Study of Health and Growth (NSHG), schools should provide separate drinking water facilities to ensure drinking water is safe (MoPHS/MoE, 2009). The findings also concur with the observations made by the researcher. The drinking points were not well maintained, some taps were faulty with dripping water making the place muddy and dirty. Sixty eight percent (68%) of the schools, with improvised points, the cans were empty because of regulation of water.

Table 4: State of Rubbish Pits as rated by respondents

	Frequency	Percentage
Poor	104	45.6
Fair	60	26.3
Good	64	28.1
Total	**228**	**100**

Source: Researcher 2016

Table 4 reveals that majority 104 (45.6%) rated the status of the rubbish pits as poor. The findings are concur with the findings of Kazungu (2017) which reported that dumpsites in schools, crumbling ceilings, cracked walls and potholed floors, characterise the conditions under which many children in public schools in Kenya learn. The observation made noted that the rubbish points available were not maintained in 45.6% of the schools and there was litter scattered all around them.

Table 5: Maintenance of sanitation facilities as rated by the respondents

Maintenance	Poor		Fair		Good	
	F	%	F	%	F	%
Toilets for boys	104	45.6	108	47.4	16	7
Toilets for girls	178	78.1	21	9.2	29	12.7
Urinals for boys	127	55.7	101	44.3	-	-
Bathrooms for girls	127	55.7	101	44.3	-	-
Handwashing for boys	149	65.4	79	34.6	-	-
Hand washing for girls	105	46.1	70	30.7	53	23.2
Drinking points	143	62.7	85	37.3	-	-
Rubbish pits	172	75.4	36	15.8	20	8.8

Table 5 reveals that a fair majority 47.4% rated the maintenance of the boys' toilets as fair. The toilets for girls were rated by 78.1% as poor while the maintenance of urinals for boys and bathrooms for girls were also rated by majority 55.7% . The findings further reveal that hand washing for boys were poorly maintained as rated by 65.4% of the respondents. This could be explained by the rough nature of boys than girls. The hand washing points for girls were however rated by 70% as fairly maintained while the drinking points were fairly maintained as rated 85% of the respondents. The study also revealed that the rubbish pits were poorly maintained as rated by 75.4% of the respondents. The findings are also in line with the findings of Mbula (2014) which recommended that school management should try and improve on maintenance, type and adequacy of sanitation facilities in their schools but give more emphasis to the adequacy of the sanitation facilities. This will ensure that all the students access the sanitation facilities without struggle.

CONCLUSION AND RECOMMENDATIONS

The study concluded that the standard of maintenance of the sanitary facilities in schools in Kericho municipality was low. Most facilities were in need of repair and maintenance. In addition, the few sanitation facilities were poorly utilized which is a result of many factors including pupils' background and up bringing, discipline regarding personal hygiene and school and weakness in implementation of sanitation and hygiene policies. For instance, key informant interviews and physical observations revealed poor disposal of solid waste especially where dustbins were ignored but disposed solid materials /waste just outside the bins yet the bins were not necessarily full. The positioning of the facilities itself is not the one recommended by the Ministry of Health.

Recommendations

1 The County government, parents and other stake holders to expand or construct more sanitation facilities to meet the increasing number of pupils and to meet the set National Standards.

REFERENCES

Barasa F.M., Wanjala C., Shaviya N, Barasa M., Sowayi .A, Vincent A., Johnston W. and Josphat O. (2015) State of sanitation and hygiene of public primary schools in Kakamega municipality, western Kenya. *International Research Journal of Public and Environmental Health* 2, (12), 215-224.

Blumende, R. S.(2001). Making schools effective in Nigeria. *Journal of Education Research,* 5(1), 65–78.

Curtis, V., Aunger, R., & Rabie, T. (2004). Evidence that disgust evolved to protect from risk of disease. *Proceedings of the Royal Society of London B: Biological Sciences, 271*(Suppl 4), S131-S133.

Gisore, A. W. (2013). *An assessment of sanitation facilities in public primary schools in Kajiado Central District* (Doctoral dissertation, University of Nairobi).
Greene et al, (2012

Hall, Andrew. (2008), A Review and Meta-Analysis of the Impact of Intestinal Worms on Child Growth and Nutrition, Maternal & Child Nutrition.
Hutton et al, 2004

IRC - International Water and Sanitation Centre (2005). *Sustainability of Hygiene Behaviour and the Effectiveness of change interventions: Lessons learned on research methodologies and research implementation from a multi-country research study.*

Kimani, B., Nyagero, J., & Ikamari, L. (2012). Knowledge, attitude and practices on jigger infestation among household members aged 18 to 60 years: case study of a rural location in Kenya. *The Pan African Medical Journal, 13* (Suppl 1).

Lilonde, R. (2004), *Scaling Up School Sanitation Promotion and Gender Concerns.* G. W. A. Netherlands.

Mbula, E. S. (2013). *Factors influencing implementation of hygiene practices in public secondary schools in central division of Machakos district in Machakos County* (Doctoral dissertation, University of Nairobi).

Oseji, M., & Okolo, A. (2011). School health services and millennium development goals. *International Journal of Collaborative Research on Internal Medicine & Public Health.*

Patton MQ. *Qualitative Research and Evaluation Methods.* Thousand Oaks, CA: Sage; 2002.

Rakungu, G. and Muthethia, D. (Amref, Jan 2006). Quality Assurance, SSHE

(www.iboro.gc.uk/well/kenya).

UNICEF (2004).*Sanitation in Uganda Schools: Stories of promise progress and challenges.* Kampala, Uganda.

UNICEF *Water, Sanitation and Hygiene Strategies* for 2000-2015. New York. (2010). *Child Friendly Schools Manual MOEST.*

United Nations (UN) (2011). *The Millennium Development Goals Report* 2011. United Nations: New York, NY, USA, 2011.

Water Aid (2013) Annual Report 2013-2014. Nepal

WHO (2010). *Reconstruction for hygiene, sanitation and water in Africa.*(1st ed.), Kampala.

World Bank.(2005), *Toolkit on hygiene, sanitation and water in schools.* World Bank: Washington DC. Retrieved from: www.schoolsanitation.com

BEI GRIN MACHT SICH IHR WISSEN BEZAHLT

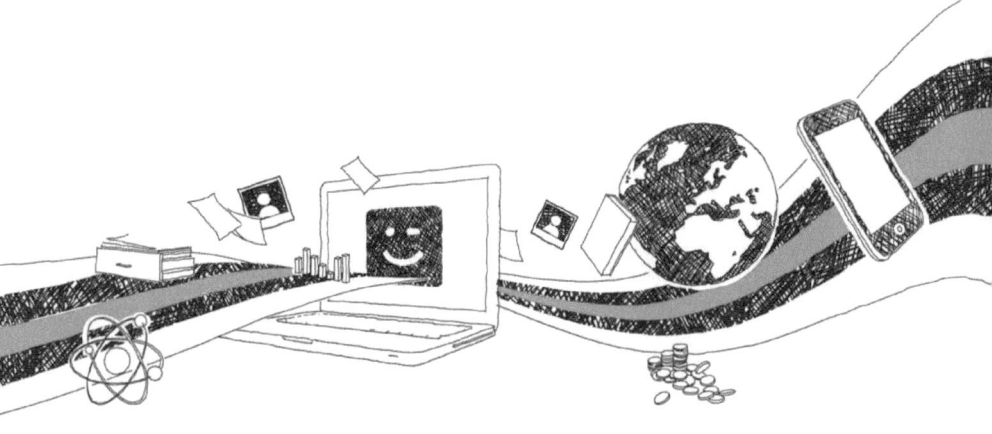

- Wir veröffentlichen Ihre Hausarbeit, Bachelor- und Masterarbeit

- Ihr eigenes eBook und Buch - weltweit in allen wichtigen Shops

- Verdienen Sie an jedem Verkauf

Jetzt bei www.GRIN.com hochladen und kostenlos publizieren

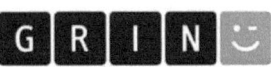